How To Get Beautiful Healthy Hair

336 Great Hair Care Tips That Everyone Should Know

ADAM COLTON

Published by BizMove
www.bizmove.com

Disclaimer

All the content found in this book was created for informational purposes only. The Content is not intended to be a substitute for professional medical advice, diagnosis, or treatment. Always seek the advice of your physician or other qualified health provider with any questions you may have regarding a medical condition. Never disregard professional medical advice or delay in seeking it because of something you have read in this book.

336 Great Hair Care Tips That Everyone Should Know

If your hair is driving you nuts, you probably just need to learn more about hair care. Learning how to take care of your hair isn't as difficult as you may think. Read on to learn what to do to take better care of your hair. You're sure to be more confident once you do.

1. If you are going to be swimming in a pool you should wet your hair beforehand so that your hair is mostly soaking up the water you put in it and not the chlorinated water. Chlorinated water is not good for your hair, especially if it is color treated.

2. People with curly hair should absolutely avoid using smoothing brushes and other brushes that have dense, fine bristles. You should use a wide-tooth comb for any combing. However, you should take care to use a heavy detangler before attempting to comb out knots and other tangles, as curly hair is susceptible to breakage.

3. Your lifestyle influences the way your hair looks. Being stressed, not getting enough sleep or smoking tobacco means your hair will not look good. You also need to maintain a balanced diet so that your

hair gets all the vitamins and nutrients it needs. Get rid of your bad habits and you should see a difference!

4. Live a healthy lifestyle for the health of your hair. Eat a balanced diet, and make sure you get plenty of exercise. Excessive smoking, not getting enough sleep, and other unhealthy habits are detrimental to the health of your hair. Take good care of yourself, and your hair will follow suit.

5. While it is practical to use a blow dryer, you should limit the amount of time that you exposure your hair to the heat that is generated from them. Always towel dry your hair as much as possible so that you will spend less time exposing it to so much heat.

6. Avoid touching your hair and scalp throughout the day. Scratching your scalp or touching your hair is going to make it more oily. If you cannot stop playing with your hair, cut it short or style it high up on your head. Once you break this bad habit, your hair should look much better.

7. To have the most luxurious hair, it all starts with eating healthy! You must eat nutritious foods, especially foods high in vitamins A and E. They help give you shiny hair! Also be sure to eat lots of

protein, as protein promotes healthy hair growth. Two great sources of protein are nuts and eggs.

8. You can use a little pomade for removing static, taming flyaways, and adding a glossy sheen to your hair. Apply a tiny amount to one hand, and then liquefy it between your palms. Afterwards, run your hands through your hair. If you are braiding, try applying it prior to braiding and then, using it for those small touch-ups.

9. Brush your hair from the scalp down to the ends to distribute the natural oils to your hair shafts. The oil in your scalp is very healthy for your hair. However, you need to get it from your scalp to your hair. You can accomplish this by brushing from the scalp to all the way down to the tips of your hair. Try bending over and brushing your hair upside down to make this a little easier to do.

10.   Do not believe the old advice about cutting your hair to encourage it to grow faster. Biologically, this is impossible. A trim can do wonders for the appearance of your hair, however, especially if the ends are split, dry or heavily damaged. For longer, healthier locks, treat your hair well and be patient as it grows.

11.   Avoid hot water when washing you hair. Lukewarm water is okay, and cold water is even better, if you can tolerate it. Hot water dries out the hair and can irritate the scalp. If you are used to a steaming hot shower, use a shower cap and wash your hair separately.

12.   A large, vented paddle brush is an excellent investment for those whose hair is very long and very thick. Taming this type of hair requires plenty of brushing. Using a paddle brush will speed up the brushing process. A vented one will help the hair dry faster, preserving its volume and bounce.

13.   Protect hair from the hot sun similarly to how you protect your skin from it. Don a scarf or hat whenever you spend time outside, or apply a styling product that contains a heat protectant. In addition to protecting your hair, it will also keep your scalp from burning from excessive exposure to the sun. Hair that is colored also fades at a faster rate with sun exposure.

14.   Try using gel for controlling hair when you desire that "wet" effect. Apply a little gel to your hair after it's styled. When braiding, use it on all of the hair prior to braiding, or when you need your hair off your face. You may even use it on the perimeter of your hairline, where the hair is shorter.

15.   Avoid using any products on your hair that contain alcohol. Some products like mousse, hairspray and gel contain alcohol which can dry hair out. If used excessively, these products can also cause damage to your hair. Before buying or using a product, check the label to be sure it doesn't contain alcohol.

16.   Never place hair products directly on the scalp. Your scalp needs to breathe if you want healthy hair, and applying these products may cause your pores to become clogged. Be careful to use these products solely on your hair to stay away from these issues.

17.   Do you suffer from dandruff? Seek out a shampoo and conditioner with an ingredient called tea tree oil! Tea tree oil is all-natural, and will work to soothe a dry scalp. This helps to prevent dandruff from being formed, and will leave your hair looking, feeling and even, smelling great.

18.   Do not style your hair with heated appliances every day. Overusing your curling iron, flat iron, blow dryer, curler or other products can cause fried, frizzy hair. Allow your hair to air-dry as often as possible, and give your hair a break from heated styling tools. If you must use these tools, apply a

heat-protective spray or balm to your hair prior to use.

19.   Women who are taller should have medium-length hair. This will make them look a little shorter than they are. On the other hand, shorter women can get away with pretty much any haircut with the exception of long hair. Shorter women tend to look even shorter when their hair is too long.

20.   Use a conditioning treatment only if your hair appears to look dry. After your hair has been washed, put on conditioner followed by your shower cap. The heat you generate will help the conditioner sink deeper into your hair strands.

21.   It is important that you only buy shampoos and conditioners that match your hair type. For example, if you have dry hair, you should purchase shampoos and conditioners made specifically for dry hair. Your hair's condition will not improve if you do not buy the relevant products to help it.

22.   Stress is one of the worst things for your body, hair and scalp as you should try to reduce this at all costs. Stress can cause dandruff and facilitate the graying process, which damages the way that you look. Eliminate stress and triggers of stress to feel and look great during the day.

23.   If you have dandruff, try using a mild shampoo. Wash your hair as often as possible and make sure that you massage your scalp. If this does not work, get an anti-dandruff shampoo. You should also look for bad habits you should get rid of, such as, not getting enough sleep.

24.   When you finish bathing, skip the blow dryer. Air drying your hair encourages volume and discourages frizz. If you must use a blow dryer, consider using it on the cool setting to encourage the sheath of your hair strands to lay down. This encourages the illusion of shine and is better for your hair than heat.

25.   Avoid touching your hair and scalp throughout the day. Scratching your scalp or touching your hair is going to make it more oily. If you cannot stop playing with your hair, cut it short or style it high up on your head. Once you break this bad habit, your hair should look much better.

26.   Choosing your shampoo and conditioner can seem overwhelming. Manufacturers spend a great deal of time and money coming up with formulas for particular hair types. Use the labels on the bottles to find the products that match your hair type. Match your conditioner to your shampoo and

try different brands, if you are unhappy with the results that you get.

27.   Check hair care products before you buy them as they may contain harmful ingredients and chemicals. Avoid alcohol in gels as it will dry your hair. Parabens, which are found in many products, have a possible link to cancer. Mineral oil may also be another carcinogen and glycerin may actually dry instead of moisturize.

28.   Protect hair from the hot sun similarly to how you protect your skin from it. You can spray your hair with sun shielding spray or put on a stylish hat to prevent the rays from reaching your hair. This also protects your scalp, which could burn. The sun also tends to fade color-treated hair a bit faster too.

29.   In the summer, refrain from staying out in the sun too long. The sun can have very damaging effects on the surface of your scalp and can also cause your hair to dry and color. Try staying indoors, as much as possible, if you desire to maintain a quality hair care regimen.

30.   If you have long hair and constantly like to wear it tied up, never, ever resort to using a plastic band for this. This item can cause serious damage and breakage, if used on a regular basis. Always buy hair

ties that have specifically designed for hair use, as these are designed to protect your follicles.

31. Avoid combing or brushing your hair when it is wet. Wet hair is most prone to damage. Try not to start brushing your hair until it is fairly dry. If you have to comb it while wet because of tangles use a wide toothed comb with tips that are round.

32. To avoid split ends, watch how you dry your hair when you get out of the bath. Vigorous drying with a towel causes the ends of the hair to split. Using the towel, gently squeeze the excess water out of your hair. To untangle any knots, use a wide-toothed comb rather than a brush.

33. Do not wash your hair immediately following having your hair colored. Wait at least a full 48 hours after getting your hair colored to wash your hair. When your hair gets wet it opens the cuticle. So it is best to leave it dry, allowing your hair to seal in the color.

34. Ensure that you get enough sleep and rest every night. A healthy amount of sleep a night is around 6-8 hours a night, depending on your body's physiology. If you get enough rest you will have a healthier body that in turn will make your hair shinier and more healthy than ever.

35.   Reduce the amount of heat you use on your hair. Hair dryers, curling irons, and flat irons can all do significant damage to your hair. Your hair and your skin aren't that different, and a product that would damage your skin will probably also damage your hair. Use these products less often or on a lower setting when possible.

36.   If you have dry hair, or just don't want to have dry hair in the future, then you want to avoid using any hair care products that contain alcohol. This is because the alcohol can make your hair even more dry. This can make your hair very brittle and easily breakable.

37.   If your hair is dry and brittle, this simple conditioning treatment is a no-brainer. Just slightly dampen your hair and use a large amount of conditioner. Wrap your hair up into a warm towel that is slightly damp. After you do this for around an hour, you should wash your hair and rinse it thoroughly.

38.   If you have oily hair, do not wash it everyday. Washing your hair two or three times a week is fine if it tends to get oily. Make sure you wash your hair thoroughly and rinse all the shampoo or conditioner

out of your hair. If your hair stays oily, try different products.

39.   When you use hair conditioner, be sure to spread it onto all areas of your hair. You should also, for best results, let the conditioner remain in your hair for a few minutes prior to rinsing it out.

40.   If your hair is often frizzy and fragile, consider cutting back on your shampoo usage. Not all types of hair require daily shampooing. Using shampoo too often can damage delicate hair. Try shampooing every other day for a week and see if your hair quality improves. Remember that rinsing your hair thoroughly is still important, even without shampoo!

41.   Coat your hair with a protective conditioner or specially-made hair wax before using heat-styling implements. Heat can dry out your hair over time, causing breakage and split ends. Some hair product manufacturers make special formulations, created for heat styling use. Typically, you just rub or spray a small amount through your hair, right before styling.

42.   Avoid touching your hair and scalp throughout the day. Scratching your scalp or touching your hair is going to make it more oily. If you cannot stop

playing with your hair, cut it short or style it high up on your head. Once you break this bad habit, your hair should look much better.

43.   To properly brush your hair, start at your ends, and work towards your scalp. Take the time to work knots out slowly so that you can avoid breaking your hair. Once they are gone, you can then brush from top to bottom carefully.

44.   Always wait until hair is dry before you brush it or comb it. Use brushed that have flexible, soft bristles, and use combs that have wide sets of teeth. If you begin at the top of your head, the tangles will accumulate as you go down, so always begin at the bottom.

45.   If you have thick, wavy, curly hair, you might want to try living without your brushes and combs. This type of hair is so dense that brushing it can often, do more harm than good. Instead, try using your fingers to comb through your hair and arrange it the way you want.

46.   In the summer, refrain from staying out in the sun too long. The sun can have very damaging effects on the surface of your scalp and can also cause your hair to dry and color. Try staying

indoors, as much as possible, if you desire to maintain a quality hair care regimen.

47.   Use beer on your hair. Beer is a great way to remove any residue or build up on your hair. Use 1 cup of warm water with 6 tablespoons of beer and after you wash and condition your hair, pour this mixture over your hair. This will help make your hair nice and shiny.

48.   Avoid getting hair products like gel, mousse or hairspray, on your scalp. These heavy products can clog your pores, limiting hair growth and sometimes acne breakouts on the scalp. Avoid all of these potential scalp and skin problems by applying these products only to your hair and not your scalp.

49.   Avoid the itchy, flaky scalp associated with dandruff by using mild shampoos and conditioners every day. Limit the use of styling products and avoid coloring or perming your hair. If dandruff persists, try an anti-dandruff shampoo for a couple of weeks. If there is still no improvement, consult a dermatologist for a medical treatment for your dry scalp.

50.   If you find that you have a knot or two in your hair, avoid brushing it at all costs. If you use a brush, you will stretch your hair and cause it to

break. For best results, pick the knot out with your fingers slowly and carefully. Be careful not to break your hair off in the process of getting the knot out.

51.   Moisturize your curly hair with natural essential oils. Regardless of ethnicity, curly hair is prone to dryness and breakage. While there are many moisturizers on the market, simple oils such as jojoba and coconut are most easily utilized by your body. Furthermore, they are inexpensive!

52.   If you can, try not to blow dry your hair too often and do not color your hair frequently. Both of these can cause your hair to dry out, damaging it in the process. If these products have already dried your hair out, you can use coconut oil twice a week to add moisture.

53.   Nevermind the old wives' tale about more frequent trims causing your hair to grow faster. Human hair tends to grow about a half-inch monthly, no matter how regularly it's cut. It may grow a bit faster during the summer, but in the end, your hormones dictate how quickly it grows, rather than how frequently you visit your stylist. A good trim will get rid of any split ends and improve your hair's appearance.

54.   Begin by combing out any tangles with a wide tooth comb starting at the ends before you use a brush on it. This will minimize any damage you do to your hair by brushing the tangles out instead of combing them. Remember to start at the ends and work your way up.

55.   While a pony tail is an easy way to style your hair when you don't have a lot of time, it's best not to style your hair this way, too often. Keeping your hair pulled back with a hair tie can lead to hair loss and damage. Be sure to change up the way you style your hair.

56.   Gently pat your hair dry with a towel rather than rubbing it violently. This can make hair frizzy and stretch it out which makes the strands break. Pat your hair dry with a towel. Also try not to brush your hair if it is wet. This can damage the ends and cause breakage.

57.   Hair should not be washed daily. If you have not had a day where your hair has gotten excessively dirty, then do not wash it. A schedule of washing every 2-3 days will prevent your hair from drying out. You will spend less time trying to rejuvenate your hair, and more time focusing on enjoying it.

58.   Limit blow dryer use. Hot air from a blow dryer can really damage your hair, so try to let it dry naturally whenever possible. If you must use one, use the lowest temperature setting and avoid letting it linger in the same spot for too long. If you towel dry your hair before you blow dry it, the hair will dry more quickly.

59.   As you compare hair care products, opt for those which are primarily made from organic or natural ingredients. Look for a conditioner and shampoo that works on your hair type. Don't hesitate to use various products to see what works best.

60.   Avoid habits that damage your body, as they will destroy your hair as well. Eating greasy foods, overwhelming stress, lack of exercise, smoking, and drinking excessively will make your body and mind ill. Your hair will reflect that by being oily or overly dry, having split ends, and dull color.

61.   Use a towel to dry your hair, as much as possible, before blow drying. When blow drying your hair, use the coolest possible setting to avoid damage. Do not leave the blow dryer in the same spot for more than a few seconds and keep it several inches away from your head.

62.　　You may find that using a deep conditioning product on a regular basis can dramatically improve the appearance of your hair. These products are designed to intensively moisturize and condition the hair, and they can produce excellent results. A weekly deep conditioning treatment will really help you out, especially if you have fine, fragile hair.

63.　　Never brush or comb your hair when it is wet unless you want to cause a lot of damage to it. If you choose a brush, look for one with natural, soft bristles. If a comb is preferred, you will have less tangles and breakage if you choose one with wide teeth and plenty of space for the hair to flow through naturally. To remove tangles, start at the ends of your hair and work your way back toward the scalp.

64.　　A large, vented paddle brush is an excellent investment for those whose hair is very long and very thick. Taming this type of hair requires plenty of brushing. Using a paddle brush will speed up the brushing process. A vented one will help the hair dry faster, preserving its volume and bounce.

65.　　When combing or brushing your hair, it is important that you use a brush with bristles that are made from animal hair. These types of brushes are softer and flexible, which will cause less harm to your hair. The less damage to your hair, the easier it will be to brush.

66.   While there are products available on the market that promise to repair split ends, there is nothing you can do that will really restore your hair back to its original state. You can apply some beeswax to it, in order to make it look better until it grows out, then the split ends should be cut off.

67.   If you are thinking about coloring your hair, you should take the time to look for a natural product. Ask your haircare specialist for advice if you need to. You should know that most products will dry your hair and weaken it. Use a special conditioner to revitalize your hair if you are going to color it.

68.   A soft, smooth pillowcase can help you keep your hairstyle, as well as, your hair. Sleeping on a pillow covered in a textured fabric or low-thread count cotton pillowcase can actually pull your hair and cause it to fall out. Use a smooth pillow-covering, wherever you lay your head and help keep your hair where it belongs.

69.   Choose shampoo, conditioner and other products, based on your hair type and needs. Colored hair benefits from UV protection and extra moisturizers, for instance. Oily hair requires a

lightweight, no-buildup conditioner. If you are unsure of your hair type, ask a cosmetologist for advice on choosing the best products for caring for your locks.

70.   It is important that you only buy shampoos and conditioners that match your hair type. For example, if you have dry hair, you should purchase shampoos and conditioners made specifically for dry hair. Your hair's condition will not improve if you do not buy the relevant products to help it.

71.   Living a healthy lifestyle has everything to do with the healthiness of your hair. Eat a balanced diet, and make sure you get plenty of exercise. Excessive smoking, not getting enough sleep, and other unhealthy habits are detrimental to the health of your hair. Take good care of yourself, and your hair will follow suit.

72.   One of the best things that you can do for your scalp and the overall health of your hair is to use leave-in conditioner. This can help to improve the texture of your hair and allows you to engage in your everyday lifestyle, without worrying about the quality of your scalp.

73.   You can have beautiful hair if you eat healthy. Since your hair is a living thing, it needs essential

nutrients to enhance its growth. Without proper nutrition, your hair may become dry, dull and prone to breakage. A significant deficiency can even cause hair loss. To keep your hair as healthy as possible be sure to consider proper nutrition.

74.   Do not forget sun protection for your hair. Over-exposure to UV rays can dry out the natural oils in your hair, leaving your hair dull, brittle, and unattractive. Be sure to wear a hat when you plan to spend a length of time in the sun. This will protect your face and your hair.

75.   If you use a blow dryer to dry your hair, be sure not to keep it on the same spot for too long. This minimizes the risk of damage to your hair due to excessive heat exposure.

76.   While friends may be an easy source for help with your hair care, make it a point to visit a professional, regularly. Though the intent of friends or acquaintances may be well-intentioned, mistakes can happen, and will often cost more to correct, than what a professional beautician would have cost you, in the first place.

77.   Do not use any settings on your blow dryer that dry your hair with heat. Heat is very damaging to your hair, especially in an effort to dry your hair

quickly. Use the cool setting, and dry your hair in a healthy manner. Doing this daily can make a big difference.

78.   You can update your style with a change in texture. You can cut down on styling time, if hair is textured. This can be achieved through a perm or by the way your hair is cut or styled. It is certainly true that the right haircut can add volume and variety to your style.

79.   You can encourage your hair to grow by brushing and combing it, because the process helps loosen and remove dead skin from the scalp. This also helps to remove dead skin which may be clogging pores and preventing healthy hair growth. Give your hair 100 brush strokes each morning, which can help stimulate the scalp to help grow hair.

80.   When you are applying conditioner to your hair, use a wide-toothed comb. This helps to distribute the conditioner evenly to all of your hair shafts. Also, the comb running through the length of the hair will help to prevent tangles. Using this method will help you have shiny, healthy-looking, tangle-free hair.

81.   People that have fine, limp strands of hair can benefit from a number of specialized products on the market. This starts with the right shampoo. If you have limpness in your hair, apply a less-is-more philosophy, otherwise you will weigh down your hair even more. This means using a volumizing shampoo and a light-weight conditioner.

82.   Your hair is a reflection of what you eat. If you notice your hair is dull and lifeless, try to cut down on the amount of cholesterol and fats in your diet. By eating healthy foods, your hair will be healthier, and in better shape. You should also drink plenty of water for your hair.

83.   Hair grows about half an inch monthly. There are some that think regular haircuts will cause hair to grow more. Most often, this is due to just having healthier hair. Frizz, split ends and other unhealthy hair makes your hair look different. A quick trim can have a powerful effect!

84.   When styling your hair, do not hesitate to go for a classic style. A complex style might not be very practical or too time-consuming. Remember that you can style your hair for different occasions and that going to work or school does not require you to spend hours on your hair.

85.   When you are washing your hair, do it in two separate steps. Take half the shampoo you would typically use for your whole head and wash your roots with that. Rinse that out, and then use some more shampoo to wash the hair shafts. This technique ensures that you wash all the hair and not just your roots.

86.   If you are looking to avoid breaking your delicate tresses, be sure to protect them when you sleep at night. Silk pillowcases are excellent for preserving hair integrity. Otherwise, you can take the time to either wrap your hair in a silk scarf, or loosely tie your hair into a low ponytail before bed.

87.   When hair conditioning, be sure to spread the conditioner evenly throughout your hair for best results. Give the conditioner a couple of minutes to soak into your hair before you rinse it out.

88.   If your hair is often frizzy and fragile, consider cutting back on your shampoo usage. Not all types of hair require daily shampooing. Using shampoo too often can damage delicate hair. Try shampooing every other day for a week and see if your hair quality improves. Remember that rinsing your hair thoroughly is still important, even without shampoo!

89.   Do not use any settings on your blow dryer that dry your hair with heat. Heat is very damaging to your hair, especially in an effort to dry your hair quickly. Use the cool setting, and dry your hair in a healthy manner. Doing this daily can make a big difference.

90.   Do not get set on a single brand of shampoo and conditioner. When you switch what brands you use every once in a while you might just see a positive reaction. Another brand may remove all the buildup and keep your scalp clean and healthy.

91.   Get a haircut every six to nine weeks to keep your hair looking its best. Over time, your hair will break and the ends will split. This creates uneven layers that make your hair look unhealthy and dull. Getting frequent haircuts will help to keep the ends from splitting all the way up to the roots, and help keep your hair shinier and healthier.

92.   Figure out what type of hair you have. The amount of times you wash your hair each week depends on the type of hair you have. If your hair is oily, you may need to shampoo and condition it every single day. On the other hand, if your hair is dry, it is recommended that you wash it every other day, at most.

93.   To improve the quality of air in your home, use a humidifier. This device can help to make the air in your home or apartment comfortable, while also restoring moisture to your hair. Keeping your hair moist is very important as you do not want it to dry out during the day.

94.   Hair products that you use to make your hair look nice can be doing more damage than you think. As you choose your products, avoid the ones that contain any alcohol. The alcohol will dry your hair out quickly. These products could also dry out your scalp, so avoid any contact with the scalp.

95.   The natural oils in your hair are there for a reason, so take care not to strip them unnecessarily when you shampoo. Though you may have naturally oily hair, applying harsh shampoos that strip oils away may in fact promote additional oiliness. Instead, choose a gentle shampoo that isn't as harmful to your hair. You can even wash with just conditioner a couple of times a week.

96.   Prior to putting on shampoo, get your hair very wet. This will help your hair stay protected, as the washing process takes place. In addition, aim to apply about a quarter-size dab of shampoo onto your head, rubbing it in your hands before putting it

on your hair. Too much shampoo could make your hair look drab and lifeless.

97.   Never use hot water on your hair. Water that is too hot can dry out even the healthiest hair, leaving it dull and lifeless. Instead, rinse with cool water after you clean your hair. Not only is the temperature easier on your locks, it will tighten up the cuticle of the hair, helping to enhance shine.

98.   As tempting as it may be, try not to get a salon perm for your hair. The chemicals that are used in perms can cause major damage to your hair, even making it fall out. If you insist on getting a perm, ask for a Acid Perm, which does not cause as much damage.

99.   If you find that your hair has split ends, you may want to try using a hot oil treatment. To do this, simply use 1/2 cup of boiling water with 1/2 cup of olive oil. Place it in a jar and apply it to your hair. Then, simply wash it out before shampooing.

100.   Outside conditions can be detrimental to your hair, but of course, you just have to make due and use other techniques that offset those complications. We all have to be outside, and everyone likes having fun in the sun. One good tip is to use a dehumidifier inside your home.

101.   Choose a hairstyle that goes well with the shape of your face. Try different styles until you find one that flatters your best features and hides the ones you do not care for. Pay attention to how people with a similar facial shape wear their hair, to get a better idea of what works and what doesn't!

102.   When you are using a hair dryer, you should take extra time to dry it on the cool setting. The cool setting on your hair dryer will cause significantly less damage to your hair, than if you dry it with very hot air. Hot air will cause drying to the hair.

103.   When you are washing your hair, do it in two separate steps. Take half the shampoo you would typically use for your whole head and wash your roots with that. Rinse that out, and then use some more shampoo to wash the hair shafts. This technique ensures that you wash all the hair and not just your roots.

104.   If you are looking to avoid breaking your delicate tresses, be sure to protect them when you sleep at night. Silk pillowcases are excellent for preserving hair integrity. Otherwise, you can take the time to either wrap your hair in a silk scarf, or loosely tie your hair into a low ponytail before bed.

105.   If you are frustrated because your hair will not grow at the rate you want it to, take a look at your diet. Your hair will not grow quickly without adequate nutritional support. Brainstorm ways that you can increase your protein intake, and minimize any junk food in your diet.

106.   You can damage your hair by blowdrying it. To minimize the harmful heat, use the lowest-temperature setting. Do not let the dryer linger on a particular area; keep it constantly moving. Get knots untangled using your fingers so you don't damage your hair later when brushing it.

107.   Try changing up the kind of shampoos and conditioners you use every now and again. Your hair may get used to the kind of products you are using and may not respond to them as well as they may have at first. Do not downgrade the brands you are using though!

108.   Don't use styling products that have alcohol in them; they can dry out hair. This is not good for your hair's health, so choose your hair care products wisely. Read the labels, and make sure the products that you purchase are good for the health of your hair.

109.   During the summer months, it's crucial that you put extra effort into caring for your hair. Always take the time to wash your hair after swimming or spending time in the sun. It's also a good idea to keep your hair covered with a bandanna or a loose cap, if you plan on being out all day.

110.   Use a towel to dry your hair, as much as possible, before blow drying. When blow drying your hair, use the coolest possible setting to avoid damage. Do not leave the blow dryer in the same spot for more than a few seconds and keep it several inches away from your head.

111.   Use two conditioners when you wash your hair. Use one in the shower after rinsing the shampoo out of your hair. The other conditioner is a leave-in conditioner. It should be applied after you are out of the shower and you towel dry your hair. The combination of conditioners will reduce the static in your hair, as well as, leaving it healthy, soft and manageable.

112.   Do not brush or comb your hair while it is wet. Hair is very fragile when it is wet, and it is important to make sure you wait until your hair is, at least, mostly dry before you comb or brush it. The brush you use should also have soft bristles.

113.   Wearing a swim cap when swimming may make you feel silly, but it is going to play a big role in how healthy your hair is. If you swim on a regular basis, you must be sure to wear the swim cap. The chlorine will damage your hair more than you could think.

114.   When drying your hair with a hair dryer, you should set it on the coolest setting. Hot air can severely damage your hair, so you do not want to keep the blow dryer blowing on one spot in your hair. Make sure you begin the drying process by patting your hair down first.

115.   If you insist upon blow drying your hair, you should do so with care. If you use a vented, wide-toothed brush and a low heat setting, you can minimize the damage you inflict on your tresses during styling. Ideally, you should keep the dryer about six inches from your head and moving at all times.

116.   Things like gel and hairspray should never be put right on the scalp. Doing this can clog up your head's pores, leading to hair growth issues, or worse, scalp pimples. Try using these products on your hair to avoid these issues.

117.   Make sure that you get enough sleep during the course of the week for the sake of your hair and scalp. Sleep is vital as it allows your body to recharge and flush out the toxins that you accumulate as the day wears on. Aim for at least eight hours of sleep for strong hair.

118.   Don't use conditioner if your hair is very greasy. If your hair is greasy, it already has enough of its own natural oils to protect it, so it does not need you to apply any artificial oils to it in the form of hair conditioner. Using hair conditioner will only make your hair even more greasy.

119.   A great hair care tip is to try out different dandruff shampoos, if you do, indeed, have dandruff. A lot of the time people with dandruff will say they aren't noticing results with their dandruff shampoo. This is because different dandruff shampoos all have different ingredients in them, so using a variety will cover all the bases.

120.   Pay attention to dry skin, especially on or near the scalp. If you have very dry skin, you may also have very dry hair. In order to combat this problem, try washing your hair only a few times a week, or using a moisturizing hair product. Avoid using heat or harsh chemicals on dry hair.

121.   Avoid using a blow dryer. The heat from a blow-dryer is often damaging to hair, so make sure to dry it naturally. Use the cool setting of your blow dryer and do not concentrate on one area of your hair very long. To quickly dry hair, dry your hair with a towel before blow drying.

122.   Buy the correct shampoo and conditioner. Only buy the type of shampoo and conditioner that is suitable for your hair type. This isn't necessarily the most expensive brand! Also, don't wash it too often or you will strip the natural oils from your hair. A good rule of thumb is every other day for oily or normal hair, and twice weekly for dry hair.

123.   To get the best shine possible to your hair, wash it with cool water. When you wash your hair with hot water, you are likely to dry out your hair in the process! Cool water, on the other hand, has the opposite effect - it can actually increase the shininess of your hair.

124.   You should get a small collection of different hair care products, including, shampoos and conditioners. Do not use the same product every time you wash your hair. Each product will affect your hair in a different way and a diverse collection of products means that your hair will never lack any vitamins.

125.   Make sure you only apply conditioner to your hair and not to your scalp. It is the hair shaft that needs to be conditioned and have the oils and moisture replaced. Applying conditioner to your scalp will only make it more oily and weigh your hair down. Start putting the conditioner on your hair from about midway down all the way to the tips.

126.   You should make sure your diet includes protein if you want your hair to look its best. Like the rest of your body, your scalp and hair require proper nutrition to stay healthy. A balanced, well-rounded diet will improve the overall quality of your hair, and including plenty of protein will make it more lustrous.

127.   Always wait at least two days to wash your hair after coloring it. When your hair has had color applied, the cuticle requires time to reseal otherwise the color will quickly fade. Even a little bit of dampness can open your hair's cuticle during the 48-hour period. By waiting a mere 48 hours you will have beautiful healthy hair.

128.   Wash your hair when it seems dirty. Some folks insist on washing their hair daily. This could cause more damage than it will help. It could cause your

hair and scalp to dry out. Typically, a person's hair only needs to be washed about two or three times a week.

129.   Avoid overusing styling products. Using too many lotions, creams, conditioners and the like can be just as destructive to the hair as using none. Hair-care products can build up over time, smothering your hair in a coating of oil and chemicals and irritating your scalp. Stick to a few reliable products and rotate them occasionally to keep them from building up.

130.   While an old wives tale states that you must brush your hair for one hundred strokes every day to achieve health, this is untrue. The only thing you will achieve by brushing this often is an overstimulated scalp that produces too much oil and makes your hair look oily and flat. Only brush until the tangles are removed.

131.   Never use hot water on your hair. Water that is too hot can dry out even the healthiest hair, leaving it dull and lifeless. Instead, rinse with cool water after you clean your hair. Not only is the temperature easier on your locks, it will tighten up the cuticle of the hair, helping to enhance shine.

132.   It is better for your hair if you wash it every other day, rather than washing it daily. Washing your hair strips it of natural oils and moisture that it needs to look shiny and stay healthy. If you must wash your hair daily, be sure that you never skip using a conditioner. The conditioner will help to replenish the moisture that is being stripped from the hair by frequent washing.

133.   Try this at home hair mask to improve the health of your hair. Start massaging some olive oil into the hair. Next, beat one egg yolk and massage it into your hair, beginning from the ends up. Leave that on for about 10 minutes, then shampoo like normal. Do this once per week for a month for best results.

134.   For the best hair possible, add massaging your scalp into your weekly routine. Massaging your scalp can loosen up and clear out dandruff and increase circulation to your head for optimum hair growth! This does not need to be done daily to be effective, once a week is enough to see great results.

135.   If you have got really dried out and damaged hair, try olive oil! At a time when you won't be going out, apply the oil in downward strokes to hair length and let it sit overnight. Olive oil will give

your hair some much needed nutrients and restore some of that luster.

136.   Do not style your hair with heated appliances every day. Overusing your curling iron, flat iron, blow dryer, curler or other products can cause fried, frizzy hair. Allow your hair to air-dry as often as possible, and give your hair a break from heated styling tools. If you must use these tools, apply a heat-protective spray or balm to your hair prior to use.

137.   Hair is very fragile when it is wet. Avoid combing or brushing your hair when it is wet. It will more easily break and stretch out when wet and you try to brush it. At the very least wait until it is damp to brush your hair out, this minimizes damage.

138.   Begin by combing out any tangles with a wide tooth comb starting at the ends before you use a brush on it. This will minimize any damage you do to your hair by brushing the tangles out instead of combing them. Remember to start at the ends and work your way up.

139.   Have a look at outside influences if you find that your hair is looking dull or flat. Factors such as nicotine, unhealthy diet, lack of physical exercise and too much stress or anxiety can all impact on the

way that your hair looks. Make changes in these areas where necessary.

140.   Use leave in conditioner on your hair on a regular basis. This is particularly useful for those who have dry and brittle hair. Using a leave in conditioner is equivalent to using a daily moisturizer on the face. It will help keep your hair healthy and replenished and prevent damage.

141.   You should make sure your diet includes protein if you want your hair to look its best. Like the rest of your body, your scalp and hair require proper nutrition to stay healthy. A balanced, well-rounded diet will improve the overall quality of your hair, and including plenty of protein will make it more lustrous.

142.   When you wash your hair, be sure to really clean your scalp. The shampoo that you use will remove the buildup of dead skin, oil, dirt and hair products that could be clogging your hair follicles. If your follicles begin to become clogged, you may start to suffer from hair loss or slowed growth.

143.   Be sure you select products that match your hair type. Everyone's hair is different, and there are many different shampooing and conditioning products to choose from. The best way to go about

doing this is by using the trial and error method. You will be able to determine which products are best for you.

144.   When combing or brushing your hair, it is important that you use a brush with bristles that are made from animal hair. These types of brushes are softer and flexible, which will cause less harm to your hair. The less damage to your hair, the easier it will be to brush.

145.   Make your hair fit your individual style. Your hair says a lot about your personality. Whether you are sophisticated and elegant, or if you like something more fun and carefree, find the right style to suit you. This will allow any first impressions you make, to be accented visually by your personality through your hairstyle.

146.   Stay away from over-brushing or over-combing your hair. Also, do not run your fingers through your hair too often. All of these things can damage fragile hair and even, make your hair fall out. Just brush, comb or finger-comb your hair, when it is absolutely necessary for you to do so.

147.   If you care about your hair, watch your stress levels. Stress can trigger a condition known as telogen effluvium, causing your hair to fall out. The

condition is usually temporary, usually dissipates as your stress levels fall. It can occur multiple times in your life, though, and in rare cases, the loss is permanent.

148.   Take the time to read the labels on all of the hair care products that you plan on using. You may find that your favorite products contain harsh chemicals or other ingredients that you'd rather not place in your hair on a consistent basis. In fact, some of these ingredients may have a short term hair benefit, but in the long run, they can damage your hair even more!

149.   Don't use a comb or a brush on wet hair. This is because your hair is extremely vulnerable while wet. Try not to start brushing your hair until it is fairly dry. If it is necessary to comb before it is dry to remove tangles, use a gentle large-tooth comb.

150.   For the best hair possible, add massaging your scalp into your weekly routine. Massaging your scalp can loosen up and clear out dandruff and increase circulation to your head for optimum hair growth! This does not need to be done daily to be effective, once a week is enough to see great results.

151.   Today there is a lot of debate over how frequently you should use shampoo. Although

skipping a day or two will not hurt your hair, neither will applying shampoo daily. Any residue that shampoo might leave in your hair is going to wash away when you rinse it. If you feel that a daily shampooing is necessary to keep your hair clean, feel free to do it.

152.   If your conditioner doesn't keep your hair as soft as it should, consider using a leave-in conditioner as well. A good leave-in conditioner can be applied right out of the shower, and will give your hair the moisture it craves. You may also want to try a deep conditioning treatment.

153.   Ensure that you get enough sleep and rest every night. A healthy amount of sleep a night is around 6-8 hours a night, depending on your body's physiology. If you get enough rest you will have a healthier body that in turn will make your hair shinier and more healthy than ever.

154.   Take a daily multi-vitamin. One of the best ways to ensure healthy hair growth is to take in a balanced diet with plenty of vitamins. Taking a daily multi-vitamin will supplement your dietary intake to ensure that your body's needs are met or exceeded. Select a high-quality vitamin designed for people of your age and gender.

155.   If you are going to be swimming in a chlorinated pool, you should make sure you wear a cap when swimming to protect it. If you do not have a cap, make sure you wash and condition your hair as soon as possible, afterwards, in order to protect it from the damage that chlorine causes.

156.   When you are washing your hair, do it in two separate steps. Take half the shampoo you would typically use for your whole head and wash your roots with that. Rinse that out, and then use some more shampoo to wash the hair shafts. This technique ensures that you wash all the hair and not just your roots.

157.   Only wash your hair as often as you think it needs washed. Everyone's hair is different but a good way to go about it is to wash it and condition it every other day or around 2-3 days a week depending on your daily activities and your body's physiology.

158.   If you have dry hair, or just don't want to have dry hair in the future, then you want to avoid using any hair care products that contain alcohol. This is because the alcohol can make your hair even more dry. This can make your hair very brittle and easily breakable.

159.   Don't use bleach on your hair. While bleach can give you great sun-kissed highlights, it also wreaks havoc with your hair structure and makes it dry and brittle. When your hair is dry and brittle, it will break easily and will be difficult to brush. Even the most expensive hair conditioners can't revive bleach damaged hair.

160.   When you brush your hair, start at the ends of your hair, then brush your way up. Work the knots out of the ends slowly and carefully to avoid any breakage. Once the tangles have been removed, one can safely brush the hair from the scalp to the ends in gentle strokes.

161.   When your hair is wet, do not use a brush or comb. Your hair is more brittle when it is wet and the comb or brush will break it severely even if you are extremely gentle. Use your figures or wide tooth pick to untangle any knots as your hair air dries.

162.   To have the most luxurious hair, it all starts with eating healthy! You must eat nutritious foods, especially foods high in vitamins A and E. They help give you shiny hair! Also be sure to eat lots of protein, as protein promotes healthy hair growth. Two great sources of protein are nuts and eggs.

163.   If you have long hair you should avoid sleeping it with in a pony tail or braid. This can cause your hair to become damaged and break off. You should either sleep with your hair loose or if you must sleep with it in a pony tail it should be a low and loose one.

164.   In the summer, refrain from staying out in the sun too long. The sun can have very damaging effects on the surface of your scalp and can also cause your hair to dry and color. Try staying indoors, as much as possible, if you desire to maintain a quality hair care regimen.

165.   If you struggle with relentlessly dry hair, consider ditching your shampoo. Curly hair, in particular, adapts remarkably well to a no-shampoo routine. You can loosen and remove dirt, dead skin and other debris as you massage your hair and scalp with conditioner instead. It may take a period of transition for the routine to begin showing full benefits, but it is worth a try for those with very dry hair and skin.

166.   Be gentle with hair that is wet. Hair that is wet is weakened because of the extra weight of the water pulling down on it. This means that wet hair is more prone to breaking. Instead of rubbing your hair with a towel to dry it, squeeze and pat instead.

This will get the water out without creating the friction that rubbing does. You should also never brush wet hair, and only use a wide-toothed comb.

167.   Though your current hairstyle may be "comfortable" for you because you have worn it for years, do not fear change. Hair styles are constantly in flux. Styles you may have overlooked because of apprehension about change, can give you a new feel and confidence, as you step out of your comfort zone.

168.   Do you want to hold your hair in place, but want a finish that is soft? Instead of spraying your hair with the hair spray, spray it into the palm of your hands and then rub it over your hair. This will give your hair a finished and soft look while controlling flyaways.

169.   Go ahead and forget the old adage about brushing your hair 100 strokes a day. Over brushing can actually lead to hair loss, breakage of strands and increased oil production. Normal brushing of your hair once or twice daily is sufficient to keep it healthy and free of tangles and build-up.

170.   Avoid damaging your hair when shampooing. Before you put any shampoo on your hair, make sure it is completely wet. Then, lather the shampoo

in your hands and apply to your hair. Scrub no longer than 30 seconds. By taking these steps, you will avoid any extra hair breakage.

171.   While you should wash your hair often, don't overdo it. Washing your hair too often, strips it of its natural oils, which gives it shine and volume. For most people, washing their hair a few times a week is enough, unless their hair is especially oily. Washing too often will turn hair dry and brittle.

172.   The idea that frequent haircuts cause your hair to grow more quickly is untrue. Human hair can grow only about half an inch every month no matter how regularly you cut it. Although, during the summer hair does tent to grow a bit faster, or if you are taking biotin supplements, but mostly it's hormones which control growth, not how often you cut it. Trims do eliminate split ends, though, which can make your hair look much better.

173.   Begin by combing out any tangles with a wide tooth comb starting at the ends before you use a brush on it. This will minimize any damage you do to your hair by brushing the tangles out instead of combing them. Remember to start at the ends and work your way up.

174.   Make sure you are getting proper nutrition and rest. Stress, on its own, does not make your hair fall out. Normal hair loss is from 50 to 120 strands each day. Stress does, however, use up additional resources and when your body becomes deficient, hair loss can result. Resources include the B Vitamins and other important nutrients. Additionally, poor sleep over time wears down your body's adrenal system, impacting hormones, which can also trigger hair loss.

175.   Use a hair serum to turn frizzy hair into hair that shines. There are many serums that have been specifically designed for whatever type of hair you may have. These serums can give your hair the sleekness and body that you are looking for. Check out your local drugstore or salong to see what they have in stock.

176.   Hair should not be washed daily. If you have not had a day where your hair has gotten excessively dirty, then do not wash it. A schedule of washing every 2-3 days will prevent your hair from drying out. You will spend less time trying to rejuvenate your hair, and more time focusing on enjoying it.

177.   If you are going to condition your hair make sure you do it directly after shampooing it. This will make sure you get the most out of your

conditioning and it will be softer and more managable than if you just shampooed it. You will have a more beautiful head of hair.

178.   Use your heat-styling implements, such as curling irons or flattening irons, on the lowest effective heat setting. Heated metal can cause your hair serious damage, especially if you have curly or dry hair. Use conditioners to lock in moisture and add strength to your hair before using these types of styling tools.

179.   You do not have to wash your hair multiple times in order for your hair to get really clean and stay very healthy. Washing your hair one time will do the trick if you take your time with the whole process and make sure that it is done thoroughly.

180.   Check hair care products before you buy them as they may contain harmful ingredients and chemicals. Avoid alcohol in gels as it will dry your hair. Parabens, which are found in many products, have a possible link to cancer. Mineral oil may also be another carcinogen and glycerin may actually dry instead of moisturize.

181.   While an old wives tale states that you must brush your hair for one hundred strokes every day to achieve health, this is untrue. The only thing you

will achieve by brushing this often is an overstimulated scalp that produces too much oil and makes your hair look oily and flat. Only brush until the tangles are removed.

182.   It is important that you never use hot water to wash your hair. The only thing this is going to do is dry your hair out and when using hot water frequently, it could even cause irreparable damage to it. It is recommended that you use lukewarm water when washing your hair.

183.   The hair will grow around a 1/2 inch per month. Some people think that trims will make your hair grow longer but it just makes it look longer and healthier. This is simply because frizz, split ends, and other damage can take away from the look of the hair. A good trim every few weeks can be very beneficial!

184.   Do you want to hold your hair in place, but want a finish that is soft? Instead of spraying your hair with the hair spray, spray it into the palm of your hands and then rub it over your hair. This will give your hair a finished and soft look while controlling flyaways.

185.   Ensure that you get enough sleep and rest every night. A healthy amount of sleep a night is around

6-8 hours a night, depending on your body's physiology. If you get enough rest you will have a healthier body that in turn will make your hair shinier and more healthy than ever.

186.   A handy tip to leave you with hair that contains no knots is to comb the conditioner through your hair with a wide-toothed comb when you are applying your conditioning treatment. This will ensure the product is spread through the hair evenly, while removing any tangles you may have at the same time.

187.   Distribute your hair's natural oils throughout all of your hair. To do this, begin by bending over and brushing your hair. Start at the scalp and brush down towards the end of your hair. Once your hair is brushed all the way through, massage your scalp with your fingers.

188.   You may be interested in trying a home remedy for dry hair. Wash your hair and wring out most of the water. Then apply conditioner liberally, put on a cap and let it sit for 10 minutes. This allows your hair to fully absorb the conditioner and lock in moisture.

189.   Begin by combing out any tangles with a wide tooth comb starting at the ends before you use a

brush on it. This will minimize any damage you do to your hair by brushing the tangles out instead of combing them. Remember to start at the ends and work your way up.

190.   Try to avoid chemicals in your hair care products, for healthier results. Many products make a lot of promises, but it's up to you to read the ingredients and determine if those promises are gimmicks or not. The more basic and natural the ingredients are, the better your results will be.

191.   Ensure that you buy shampoos and conditioners that are made specifically for your hair type. This will ensure that you will be getting the most out of your hair cleaning products and not weighing it down with heavier products, if you do not need them. Your hair will thank you!

192.   If you are frustrated because your hair will not grow at the rate you want it to, take a look at your diet. Your hair will not grow quickly without adequate nutritional support. Brainstorm ways that you can increase your protein intake, and minimize any junk food in your diet.

193.   A great way that you can reduce the breakage of your hair is to put tea tree oil in your shampoo. This nutrient is very important for the health of your hair

and helps to maintain firm strands. Adding this nutrient to your shampoo or conditioner yields a fresh and vibrant style.

194.   If your hair has become dull, you may need to use a clarifying shampoo. You can obtain dull hair from buildup of other hair products used in your hair. To avoid such a result, use clarifying shampoos on a weekly basis as a means to remove excess dirt and product residue.

195.   Only wash your hair as often as you think it needs washed. Everyone's hair is different but a good way to go about it is to wash it and condition it every other day or around 2-3 days a week depending on your daily activities and your body's physiology.

196.   When you wash your hair, be sure to really clean your scalp. The shampoo that you use will remove the buildup of dead skin, oil, dirt and hair products that could be clogging your hair follicles. If your follicles begin to become clogged, you may start to suffer from hair loss or slowed growth.

197.   Before blow drying your hair, towel-dry it thoroughly. This will not only save you time when drying your hair, but it will also keep your hair in better shape. By using less heat on your hair, you

will be avoiding extra damage by using too much heat used to get your hair dry.

198.   Don't use salt spray on your hair. While salt spray is great for creating beach waves and minimizing grease on your hair, it is also very damaging to your hair. After all, salt is a drying agent, so it will take all of the moisture out of your hair and leave it dry and brittle.

199.   Limit your sun exposure. It is widely known that the sun's rays are harmful to your skin; however they can be just as harmful to your hair as well. The ultraviolet radiation can weaken your hair on its own, and if it is combined with harsh pool chemicals, such as chlorine, the effects can be devastating.

200.   Wash your hair 3-4 times per week at most if you have hair that is curly. To keep your hair from tangling, you'll want to apply a specially-formulated conditioner on it before it dries. Stay away from blow dryers that will lead to frizzy hair.

201.   If you have long hair and constantly like to wear it tied up, never, ever resort to using a plastic band for this. This item can cause serious damage and breakage, if used on a regular basis. Always buy hair

ties that have specifically designed for hair use, as these are designed to protect your follicles.

202.   Put a leave-in conditioner in your hair if you must use a blow dryer. When you blow dry your hair, the conditioner will keep your hair from falling out and getting dry and brittle. Of course, it's best to just keep away from blow drying altogether, unless you really have to.

203.   You should try to wear a cap when swimming in pools whenever possible, in order to protect your hair from the chlorine that is added. If you do not wear a cap when swimming, you should make sure to wash your hair and then, condition it, right after you are done.

204.   You can revive parched tresses using ingredients in your cupboard. When your hair has been washed and you have somewhat dried it, add conditioner and a shower cap onto it for several minutes. This way, heat is generated and the conditioner is able to get further into your hair follicles.

205.   Choose shampoo, conditioner and other products, based on your hair type and needs. Colored hair benefits from UV protection and extra moisturizers, for instance. Oily hair requires a lightweight, no-buildup conditioner. If you are

unsure of your hair type, ask a cosmetologist for advice on choosing the best products for caring for your locks.

206.   If you have curly hair, put down the brush and comb! Curly hair should only be brushed or combed while it is soaking wet. For the best results, apply conditioner to your wet hair before you comb through it. Be sure to only use a wide toothed comb so as to not cause any damage. This will keep your curls looking their best.

207.   When you are in the shower and washing your hair, make sure you turn your hot water down, whenever you are doing your washing and conditioning. Hot water can dry out and irritate your scalp and this can cause flaking and dandruff that is unattractive and also, hard to get rid of.

208.   Take care of your hair during the summer. Over exposure to sun and chlorine can seriously damage hair and result in split ends. Wear a hat in the sun, and a latex swim cap while in the pool. Also, wash your hair with a chlorine-removal shampoo in fresh water after swimming in a chlorinated pool.

209.   If you have dull hair, you should try a clarifying shampoo. Hair that is dull can be caused by hair care product build up. In order to prevent this, you

should use some kind of clarifying shampoo once or twice per week to eliminate built-up dirt or residue.

210.   Use products that have natural ingredients when you use hair care products. In addition, you need to search for shampoos and conditioners that are appropriate for your particular hair type. You may need to try a variety of products before finding ones that you like; that's fine.

211.   It is not true that if you pluck out one gray hair, several will grow in its place. It is true, however, that you could damage the hair's root, cause an infection or leave scarring if you pluck out gray hairs. Additionally, as can be seen in over-plucked eyebrows, when you pluck out hair, it does not always grow back.

212.   Stay away from being too brand loyal on shampoos and conditioners. By altering the brands that are being used on a semi-regular basis, your hair will be jolted into a positive reaction. One brand may remove the buildup of another and keep the scalp healthy and clean.

213.   To protect your hair from sun damage, it may be wise to wear a hat or other head covering if you know you are going to be the sun for an extended

period of time. The sun causes your hair to dry out and damage, which is why it is crucial that you protect it.

214.   You do not have to wash your hair multiple times in order for your hair to get really clean and stay very healthy. Washing your hair one time will do the trick if you take your time with the whole process and make sure that it is done thoroughly.

215.   When combing or brushing your hair, it is important that you use a brush with bristles that are made from animal hair. These types of brushes are softer and flexible, which will cause less harm to your hair. The less damage to your hair, the easier it will be to brush.

216.   Try using gel for controlling hair when you desire that "wet" effect. Apply a little gel to your hair after it's styled. When braiding, use it on all of the hair prior to braiding, or when you need your hair off your face. You may even use it on the perimeter of your hairline, where the hair is shorter.

217.   Choose silk over cotton. Cotton pillowcases can be bad for long hair because it causes breaks and damage to your hair when it catches on the corners, etc. This happens if you toss and turn during the

night. Try buying a silk pillowcase to minimize the amount of damage the pillowcase may do.

218. Stay away from over-brushing or over-combing your hair. Also, do not run your fingers through your hair too often. All of these things can damage fragile hair and even, make your hair fall out. Just brush, comb or finger-comb your hair, when it is absolutely necessary for you to do so.

219. Although you can save some money doing highlighting, dyeing, and perming at home, you'll find that you get much better results if you let a professional handle these hair styling tasks. Home kits can do a great deal of damage to your hair, and undoing that damage can be quite costly. A good professional hair stylist will give you the hair you desire without the damage.

220. Avoid damaging your hair when shampooing. Before you put any shampoo on your hair, make sure it is completely wet. Then, lather the shampoo in your hands and apply to your hair. Scrub no longer than 30 seconds. By taking these steps, you will avoid any extra hair breakage.

221. Do you suffer from dandruff? Seek out a shampoo and conditioner with an ingredient called tea tree oil! Tea tree oil is all-natural, and will work

to soothe a dry scalp. This helps to prevent dandruff from being formed, and will leave your hair looking, feeling and even, smelling great.

222.   When choosing a brush to use on your hair, choose one with soft bristles, instead of hard ones. There are brushes available that are made of animal fibers or soft bristles that will be easier on your hair and not cause any type of damage to your beautiful hair!

223.   When you are in the shower and washing your hair, make sure you turn your hot water down, whenever you are doing your washing and conditioning. Hot water can dry out and irritate your scalp and this can cause flaking and dandruff that is unattractive and also, hard to get rid of.

224.   A balanced diet full of protein, vitamin and minerals is the best way to make sure your hair stays healthy. To look beautiful, your hair needs a healthy diet. A deficiency in any combination of nutrients can lead to weak, brittle and unattractive hair. An extremely poor diet can even cause your hair to fall out. Eat properly if you want healthy hair.

225.   When selecting a brush, you should choose one that is made from natural animal hairs, as opposed to one made from synthetic materials. The bristles

on the natural brushes will be more soft and flexible, so it will be less likely to cause any damage to your hair, if you use it regularly.

226.   Do not forget sun protection for your hair. Over-exposure to UV rays can dry out the natural oils in your hair, leaving your hair dull, brittle, and unattractive. Be sure to wear a hat when you plan to spend a length of time in the sun. This will protect your face and your hair.

227.   To keep your hair from getting dried out, avoid any hair care product that includes alcohol in its list of ingredients. Take some time to learn about the products you use, as they are not all good for you simply because they can be purchased in a store. Read labels, and be certain the products you buy will benefit your hair.

228.   If you are going to condition your hair make sure you do it directly after shampooing it. This will make sure you get the most out of your conditioning and it will be softer and more managable than if you just shampooed it. You will have a more beautiful head of hair.

229.   Avoid spending too much time outdoors during the coldest months. Cold weather dries out hair, reducing the amount of natural oils that keep your

hair healthy and lubricated. If you need to stay outdoors for a long time, make sure to wear a hat.

230.   Chlorinated water can be extremely damaging to your hair, but everyone still needs to have fun and go swimming right? Here is what you do. Wet your hair thoroughly before you get in the pool, so your hair soaks up that water, instead of the chlorinated water. This is much better for the health of your hair.

231.   Figure out what type of hair you have. The amount of times you wash your hair each week depends on the type of hair you have. If your hair is oily, you may need to shampoo and condition it every single day. On the other hand, if your hair is dry, it is recommended that you wash it every other day, at most.

232.   You shouldn't use hair products with alcohol in them, because these can dry out your hair. Also, do not apply products directly to your scalp, to avoid irritation or clogged pores. Both of these can lead to unhealthy hair.

233.   You must drink lots of water to have the healthiest hair possible. Water not only hydrates your body, it also hydrates your hair. Drinking plenty of water makes sure that your hair is

hydrated, which leads to less frizzy days! As a goal, always try to drink about eight glasses of water every day.

234.   When drying your hair with a hair dryer, you should set it on the coolest setting. Hot air can severely damage your hair, so you do not want to keep the blow dryer blowing on one spot in your hair. Make sure you begin the drying process by patting your hair down first.

235.   Though it may seem a bit more costly, stick with professional-grade hair care products. Generic or low-price, low-quality products can leave you wondering what all the promises on the bottle are about. Professional level products are designed to maximize benefits with each use. If cost is a concern, look for specials on the quality products.

236.   If you are interested in going blond, try highlights first! Lightening your hair to the extreme can cause serious damage, so be sure it's something you really want before committing to it. Pretty highlights might be just the thing that you need to brighten your hair, without the harsh damage that coloring can do.

237.   When you are using a hair dryer, you should take extra time to dry it on the cool setting. The cool

setting on your hair dryer will cause significantly less damage to your hair, than if you dry it with very hot air. Hot air will cause drying to the hair.

238.   When selecting a brush, you should choose one that is made from natural animal hairs, as opposed to one made from synthetic materials. The bristles on the natural brushes will be more soft and flexible, so it will be less likely to cause any damage to your hair, if you use it regularly.

239.   Take care of your hair during the summer. Over exposure to sun and chlorine can seriously damage hair and result in split ends. Wear a hat in the sun, and a latex swim cap while in the pool. Also, wash your hair with a chlorine-removal shampoo in fresh water after swimming in a chlorinated pool.

240.   To get the best shine possible to your hair, wash it with cool water. When you wash your hair with hot water, you are likely to dry out your hair in the process! Cool water, on the other hand, has the opposite effect - it can actually increase the shininess of your hair.

241.   Focus on hair color products that contain conditioners and cause little damage. Though you may find inexpensive solutions for coloring your hair, the lack of conditioners could leave your hair

strained and lifeless. The recuperation efforts that you will put into your hair after coloring will be reduced when conditioners are incorporated.

242.	Make sure you only apply conditioner to your hair and not to your scalp. It is the hair shaft that needs to be conditioned and have the oils and moisture replaced. Applying conditioner to your scalp will only make it more oily and weigh your hair down. Start putting the conditioner on your hair from about midway down all the way to the tips.

243.	A satin pillowcase can be used if you want to protect your curly hair at night. Cotton pillowcases absorb the oil and moisture from your hair. Satin pillowcases protect your hair making you wake up having the same types of curls when you slept. You can get the same effect by wearing a scarf or bonnet of satin to bed, too.

244.	When you wash your hair, be sure to really clean your scalp. The shampoo that you use will remove the buildup of dead skin, oil, dirt and hair products that could be clogging your hair follicles. If your follicles begin to become clogged, you may start to suffer from hair loss or slowed growth.

245.   Don't use bleach on your hair. While bleach can give you great sun-kissed highlights, it also wreaks havoc with your hair structure and makes it dry and brittle. When your hair is dry and brittle, it will break easily and will be difficult to brush. Even the most expensive hair conditioners can't revive bleach damaged hair.

246.   Do not believe the old advice about cutting your hair to encourage it to grow faster. Biologically, this is impossible. A trim can do wonders for the appearance of your hair, however, especially if the ends are split, dry or heavily damaged. For longer, healthier locks, treat your hair well and be patient as it grows.

247.   Like your skin, your hair should be protected against damage from sun exposure. Always use a hat or spray that protects your hair when you are outdoors in the sun and wind. As an added benefit you will be protecting your scalp from the damage caused by the sun. Hair that is color-treated usually fades quicker in the sun, too.

248.   If you are thinking about coloring your hair, you should take the time to look for a natural product. Ask your haircare specialist for advice if you need to. You should know that most products will dry

your hair and weaken it. Use a special conditioner to revitalize your hair if you are going to color it.

249.   If you value your hair color, wear a swimming cap before jumping into a chlorinated pool. Chlorine causes hard metals, present in all water in various concentrations, to oxidize, and that in turn can add a green tinge to any hair color. Applying a coat of conditioner before swimming can help, but most public pools frown on that practice. Stick to swimming in lakes and ponds to keep hair from looking like it belongs on a Martian.

250.   Make your hair fit your individual style. Your hair says a lot about your personality. Whether you are sophisticated and elegant, or if you like something more fun and carefree, find the right style to suit you. This will allow any first impressions you make, to be accented visually by your personality through your hairstyle.

251.   Try this at home hair mask to improve the health of your hair. Start massaging some olive oil into the hair. Next, beat one egg yolk and massage it into your hair, beginning from the ends up. Leave that on for about 10 minutes, then shampoo like normal. Do this once per week for a month for best results.

252. Never brush your hair when it is wet. Wet hair is most prone to damage. Be sure that your hair is almost all the way dry prior to brushing it. Wet hair is tangled hair, and people have a propensity to tug and pull on tangles and thus damage their hair. So, avoid wet combing!

253. Avoid damaging your hair when shampooing. Before you put any shampoo on your hair, make sure it is completely wet. Then, lather the shampoo in your hands and apply to your hair. Scrub no longer than 30 seconds. By taking these steps, you will avoid any extra hair breakage.

254. Heavy conditioners are not meant for fine, thin hair. This will make your hair look finer and thinner and weigh it down. If you'd like to add a little volume without weighing down your hair, try using a light leave-in conditioner or a conditioning mousse.

255. The myth that getting your hair trimmed regularly makes it grow faster is false. It doesn't matter how much you cut it, hair grows at about half an inch a month. Your hair may grow a little faster during the summer months or if you use biotin supplements. The main driver of hair growth is hormones; your stylist has nothing to do with it.

A simple trim will get rid of split ends, which does give your hair a much better look.

256. Using hair care products that have sunscreen in them can protect your hair from sun damage. Too much sun can damage your hair and make it harder to care for. When you take steps to keep your hair protected, it will have longevity and will be less likely to lighten in color.

257. If you have curly hair, put down the brush and comb! Curly hair should only be brushed or combed while it is soaking wet. For the best results, apply conditioner to your wet hair before you comb through it. Be sure to only use a wide toothed comb so as to not cause any damage. This will keep your curls looking their best.

258. Use a hair serum to turn frizzy hair into hair that shines. There are many serums that have been specifically designed for whatever type of hair you may have. These serums can give your hair the sleekness and body that you are looking for. Check out your local drugstore or salong to see what they have in stock.

259. If you are going to condition your hair make sure you do it directly after shampooing it. This will make sure you get the most out of your

conditioning and it will be softer and more managable than if you just shampooed it. You will have a more beautiful head of hair.

260.   If you have dandruff, try using a mild shampoo. Wash your hair as often as possible and make sure that you massage your scalp. If this does not work, get an anti-dandruff shampoo. You should also look for bad habits you should get rid of, such as, not getting enough sleep.

261.   To prevent nighttime damage to your hair, use a satin pillowcase. Cotton pillowcases absorb the oil and moisture from your hair. Satin pillowcases will protect hair, and let you wake in the morning with similar curls to the ones you slept with. A satin nightcap or scarf will also work to protect your curls.

262.   Before blow drying your hair, towel-dry it thoroughly. This will not only save you time when drying your hair, but it will also keep your hair in better shape. By using less heat on your hair, you will be avoiding extra damage by using too much heat used to get your hair dry.

263.   When you see gray hair start to appear on your head, you should not pluck them. Most people believe that it's because two will grow back in its

place, but the real reason is because you can damage the root of your hair by pulling it out. That could lead to an infection at some point.

264.   People whose hair is naturally frizzy or coarse need to use a good moisturizing mask product more frequently than others. In general, such products should be applied every two to four weeks. Those with frizzy hair that is susceptible to drying out will want to apply a mask every week to keep their hair smooth and moisturized.

265.   Limit your sun exposure. It is widely known that the sun's rays are harmful to your skin; however they can be just as harmful to your hair as well. The ultraviolet radiation can weaken your hair on its own, and if it is combined with harsh pool chemicals, such as chlorine, the effects can be devastating.

266.   Treating your hair from the inside out is the best way to achieve the look that you desire during the day. Make sure that you drink and eat a lot of fruit and vegetables, which are packed with antioxidants. These foods can help to reduce toxins in your body, yielding a healthy scalp.

267.   If you find yourself free of dandruff after using a shampoo for that purpose, keep on using it. If you

stop using that shampoo, it is likely that dandruff could reoccur because of the fact that there is no cure for dandruff. The shampoo you are using is keeping it away, so you should keep using it.

268.   In order to keep your hair healthy and looking its best, try cutting back on the amount of blow drying you do. No matter how carefully you go about it, blow drying your hair will cause some damage to it. Giving your hair a break from frequent styling can help it recuperate and return to its full, natural potential.

269.   When you are attending to the shampooing and conditioning of your hair, make sure that you thoroughly rinse off all product after it has been applied and that none remains on your hair follicles. Product that is left to build up on your hair can lead to lifeless and dull locks.

270.   You should try to wear a cap when swimming in pools whenever possible, in order to protect your hair from the chlorine that is added. If you do not wear a cap when swimming, you should make sure to wash your hair and then, condition it, right after you are done.

271.   When drying your hair with a blow dryer, continuously wave the blow dryer back and forth so

the hot air it produces doesn't blow on one section of your hair too long. This can reduce the amount of damage that heat can cause.

272.   If you are going to condition your hair make sure you do it directly after shampooing it. This will make sure you get the most out of your conditioning and it will be softer and more managable than if you just shampooed it. You will have a more beautiful head of hair.

273.   Keep your hair care tools clean. Use shampoo or body soap to clean them each week. It will keep your hair cleaner as you brush it. Use a comb to clean your brushes out thoroughly. Make sure to rinse them thoroughly and allow them to dry completely before using them.

274.   To improve the quality of air in your home, use a humidifier. This device can help to make the air in your home or apartment comfortable, while also restoring moisture to your hair. Keeping your hair moist is very important as you do not want it to dry out during the day.

275.   Be sure you select products that match your hair type. Everyone's hair is different, and there are many different shampooing and conditioning products to choose from. The best way to go about

doing this is by using the trial and error method. You will be able to determine which products are best for you.

276.   Overall, living a healthy lifestyle will keep your hair happy. Make sure you get enough exercise, drink plenty of water daily, and avoid stress and bad habits like smoking. These types of things, along with plenty of rest, can make a huge difference.

277.   You may think it counter-intuitive, but your hair is the most delicate when it is wet. Avoid brushing and combing your hair until it has dried fully. Otherwise, your hair will look frizzy, dull, and angry. Furthermore, you risk extensive damage and breakage when brushing your hair while it is wet.

278.   If you have dry hair, you might want to use cooler water when you shower. Hot water can dry your hair and scalp, which creates a host of problems. Warm water is a much better alternative as it is easier on your body. And, for a little shine, a blast of cool water after shampooing should do the trick!

279.   If you have very dry hair, you should deep condition it. You can do this deep conditioning treatment at home if your hair is brittle and dry. All you have to do is dampen clean hair. Use a thick

conditioner, then work it through your hair in a thorough manner. Next, seal your hair in a plastic cap, and let your hair soak for half an hour. Finish by thoroughly rinsing all traces of product from your hair; you should immediately notice softer, more healthy hair.

280.   Something that is not recommended is brushing your hair all the time. Brushing your hair can keep it manageable and soft, but overdoing it can do more damage than good. Individual hairs can get damaged by over-brushing, and doing too much of it will yank hairs right out of their follicles.

281.   Take the time to read the labels on all of the hair care products that you plan on using. You may find that your favorite products contain harsh chemicals or other ingredients that you'd rather not place in your hair on a consistent basis. In fact, some of these ingredients may have a short term hair benefit, but in the long run, they can damage your hair even more!

282.   Make sure that you use hair care products that are formulated for your specific hair type. Using the wrong type can cause damage to your hair. For example, using a product that is made for people with oily hair may remove oils from the head of a

person with brittle hair, which would cause damage and/or hair loss.

283.   Avoid the itchy, flaky scalp associated with dandruff by using mild shampoos and conditioners every day. Limit the use of styling products and avoid coloring or perming your hair. If dandruff persists, try an anti-dandruff shampoo for a couple of weeks. If there is still no improvement, consult a dermatologist for a medical treatment for your dry scalp.

284.   To avoid split ends, watch how you dry your hair when you get out of the bath. Vigorous drying with a towel causes the ends of the hair to split. Using the towel, gently squeeze the excess water out of your hair. To untangle any knots, use a wide-toothed comb rather than a brush.

285.   Create a moisturizing hair treatment using mayonnaise and egg. These two ingredients can add shine, volume, and bounce back into your hair. Simply blend an egg (or two if you have long hair) with a little mayonnaise to create a cream. Work it into your hair, starting at the scalp and moving down towards the ends and leave it in for 15 minutes. Once the time is up, shampoo and condition as you normally would. This treatment can be repeated every week for luxurious locks.

286.   For minimizing breakage, be sure that your hair is completely wet prior to applying shampoo. Don't use any more than about a quarter-size dollop. Then proceed to rub the shampoo in between your palms to start with. Be sure to lather up for no more than 30 seconds or so.

287.   Try to not use your blow dryer frequently. Let your hair dry on its own rather than damaging it with too much hot air. If you must use one, use the lowest temperature setting and avoid letting it linger in the same spot for too long. You can dry your hair faster if you use a towel to dry before blowing it dry.

288.   To avoid damaging your hair while blow drying, do not leave blow dryer in one area for too long. Concentrating on one area makes your hair more prone to heat damage.

289.   Be sure to select a hair style that works with your face shape. A hair cut may look fantastic on your friend or a celebrity, but that doesn't mean it'll flatter you. Find a hair stylist you can work with, and come up with a hair cut that will make your features shine.

290.   Make sure you only apply conditioner to your hair and not to your scalp. It is the hair shaft that needs to be conditioned and have the oils and moisture replaced. Applying conditioner to your scalp will only make it more oily and weigh your hair down. Start putting the conditioner on your hair from about midway down all the way to the tips.

291.   Sometimes, you may be allergic to something in the air, which can affect the quality of your hair. Take a ride to the doctor's to see if there is something airborne that is affecting your health or physical characteristics. This can help to nip the problem in the bud, so that it doesn't become a more serious issue.

292.   Keep in mind that aging results in normal hair changes. It is natural for hair to lose some moisture, to change texture and to go gray. It may even change textures, such as becoming curly or straight. Speak with your doctor if you are having difficult issues with your hair and its texture.

293.   Your hair is a reflection of what you eat. If you notice your hair is dull and lifeless, try to cut down on the amount of cholesterol and fats in your diet. By eating healthy foods, your hair will be healthier,

and in better shape. You should also drink plenty of water for your hair.

294.   Use water to perk up your curls. If your curls tend to fall between shampoos, mist your hair lightly with water. Once your hair is slightly damp, curl your hair with your fingers. This will help add some pep to your curls until the next time you shampoo your hair.

295.   If you struggle with relentlessly dry hair, consider ditching your shampoo. Curly hair, in particular, adapts remarkably well to a no-shampoo routine. You can loosen and remove dirt, dead skin and other debris as you massage your hair and scalp with conditioner instead. It may take a period of transition for the routine to begin showing full benefits, but it is worth a try for those with very dry hair and skin.

296.   Although there is no permanent solution for split ends, products are available that can temporarily minimize the problem. These products work by "gluing" split ends back together. Always keep in mind that this is a temporary solution and using these products frequently will not cure split ends. It can even cause additional damage to the hair.

297.   Avoid using hot air to dry your hair. Hot air can cause damage to your hair. If you must blow dry your hair, use the cool setting. Many new hair dryers have this setting. This will still dry your hair, but it won't cause the damage that hot air causes.

298.   Do not brush or comb your hair when it is wet. The most damage occurs when your hair is wet. Don't start brushing your hair until it's almost completely dry. If you have to comb it while wet because of tangles use a wide toothed comb with tips that are round.

299.   Those with curly hair ought to restrict themselves to two washes per week. Shampooing can strip natural oils from the hair which hair needs to appear shiny and healthy. It is very important to make sure that you thoroughly rinse all shampoo residue from you hair.

300.   Though your current hairstyle may be "comfortable" for you because you have worn it for years, do not fear change. Hair styles are constantly in flux. Styles you may have overlooked because of apprehension about change, can give you a new feel and confidence, as you step out of your comfort zone.

301.   Do you want to hold your hair in place, but want a finish that is soft? Instead of spraying your hair with the hair spray, spray it into the palm of your hands and then rub it over your hair. This will give your hair a finished and soft look while controlling flyaways.

302.   Today there is a lot of debate over how frequently you should use shampoo. Although skipping a day or two will not hurt your hair, neither will applying shampoo daily. Any residue that shampoo might leave in your hair is going to wash away when you rinse it. If you feel that a daily shampooing is necessary to keep your hair clean, feel free to do it.

303.   If your conditioner doesn't keep your hair as soft as it should, consider using a leave-in conditioner as well. A good leave-in conditioner can be applied right out of the shower, and will give your hair the moisture it craves. You may also want to try a deep conditioning treatment.

304.   Ensure that you get enough sleep and rest every night. A healthy amount of sleep a night is around 6-8 hours a night, depending on your body's physiology. If you get enough rest you will have a healthier body that in turn will make your hair shinier and more healthy than ever.

305.   If you plan on going swimming you should wet your hair before entering the pool. Most pool water has chlorine in it and it can cause damage to hair. Wetting the hair before going in will ensure that your hair soak up fresh water instead of the chlorine filled water in the pool.

306.   You should try to wear a cap when swimming in pools whenever possible, in order to protect your hair from the chlorine that is added. If you do not wear a cap when swimming, you should make sure to wash your hair and then, condition it, right after you are done.

307.   When choosing your hair products, look for products with no alcohol. Applying alcohol on your hair will make it very dry and fragile. If you still want to use products containing alcohol, avoid using these products on a daily basis and wash your hair thoroughly afterward, so that the product is rinsed out.

308.   Products containing sunscreen can help prevent sun damage. The sun can be damaging to your hair and eliminate any benefits you may gain from your care routine. By taking additional measures to protect your hair, you ensure that it looks and feels great and retains its color.

309.   One of the best things that you can do for your scalp and the overall health of your hair is to use leave-in conditioner. This can help to improve the texture of your hair and allows you to engage in your everyday lifestyle, without worrying about the quality of your scalp.

310.   Regardless of how you feel about shampooing, you ought to make it a habit to use conditioner every day. Conditioner is one of the most powerful tools in your hair-care arsenal. It can repair everyday wear and tear and restore your hair to its natural strength and shininess. Be extra certain to condition your hair daily during the winter months.

311.   When combing or brushing the hair, it is important to begin at the ends of your hair, and detangle your way upwards toward your scalp. Go slow and take care not to rip or tear the delicate strands of your hair. As you work the knots out, you can then use complete strokes from the roots to tips slowly and gently.

312.   To keep your hair from breaking, don't brush or comb your locks until they're dry. Use a brush with soft, flexible bristles and a comb with wide set teeth. Start combing the tangles from the ends of your hair and work your way up to the scalp.

313.   One of the things that you can do during the day to restore blood flow in your scalp is to give your head a massage. This procedure can also help to reduce drying of your hair, as you are keeping your head and scalp active. Rub your hands slowly through your hair, in order to improve your overall hair health.

314.   Avoid hot water when washing you hair. Lukewarm water is okay, and cold water is even better, if you can tolerate it. Hot water dries out the hair and can irritate the scalp. If you are used to a steaming hot shower, use a shower cap and wash your hair separately.

315.   Keep in mind that the hair changes as you age. As you age, your hair normally becomes drier, more brittle and begins to turn gray. You may even experience a texture change, like curly to straight, or vice versa. It is, however, a good idea to consult a doctor if your hair texture changes unexpectedly or in a way that concerns you.

316.   It is a widespread myth that using a coloring product on the hair will always leave the hair damaged and weakened. Most coloring products these days are formulated with a lot of added

conditioners so it is pretty safe to use them. Go to a salon if you are not sure of how to do it.

317.   If you suffer from dry hair, take a warm shower instead of a hot shower. Scalding hot water is damaging to both your hair, and your scalp. Warm water is much better for your hair and your body. For some extra shine, rinse your hair with cold water after your hair is clean.

318.   To have the healthiest hair possible, stay away from exposing it to harsh chemicals. This includes exposure to hair-relaxing solutions (often lye-based), heat-styling products, alcohol based products, and even the chlorine in swimming pools. With prolonged exposures, these chemicals can really take the shine right out of your hair.

319.   Choose silk over cotton. Cotton pillowcases can be bad for long hair because it causes breaks and damage to your hair when it catches on the corners, etc. This happens if you toss and turn during the night. Try buying a silk pillowcase to minimize the amount of damage the pillowcase may do.

320.   For those with curly hair, nix SLS (sodium lauryl sulfate) from your hair care routine, for bouncy, care-free curls. SLS is a harsh stripping agent that robs your hair of essential oils. This creates the

illusion of frizz and encourages breakage. You can spot this substance by checking the ingredients of your products.

321. If you are going to be swimming in a pool you should wet your hair before hand so that your hair is mostly soaking up the water you put in it and not the chlorinated water. Chlorinated water is not good for your hair, especially if it is color treated.

322. For a quick and easy on the go hair tamer, try a dab of your favorite hand lotion. Simply rub a small amount into the palm of your hand and stroke your hair in a downward direction. This will tame frizz instantly and even offer the benefit of conditioning your hair, as well.

323. It is crucial that you get a haircut every 5 to 6 weeks. This is because human hair grows about a quarter to a half an inch every month, and when hair grows, split ends tend to form. Getting a haircut this frequently will prevent split ends from occurring, while getting rid of any you may have.

324. Use a soft brush made out of animal hairs instead of plastic. Do not brush your hair when it is wet and always be gentle. You should start at the end of your hair and work your way up as you

gently untangle all the knots. Make sure you take your time!

325.   Do not use any settings on your blow dryer that dry your hair with heat. Heat is very damaging to your hair, especially in an effort to dry your hair quickly. Use the cool setting, and dry your hair in a healthy manner. Doing this daily can make a big difference.

326.   Do not brush or comb your hair while it is wet. Hair is very fragile when it is wet, and it is important to make sure you wait until your hair is, at least, mostly dry before you comb or brush it. The brush you use should also have soft bristles.

327.   A healthy diet will show in your hair. If you eat a diet high in fat and cholesterol, your hair may appear dull and lifeless. For healthier hair, a well-balanced diet is best. Eat food that is low in fat and cholesterol, and high in anti-oxidants, protein, vitamins and minerals.

328.   If you are an avid swimmer or simply take a dip in the pool from time to time, try using a swimming cap to prevent chlorine from touching your hair. Chlorine can negatively impact your scalp and cause drying, which is something that you want to avoid, especially in the colder seasons.

329.   To have the healthiest hair possible, stay away from exposing it to harsh chemicals. This includes exposure to hair-relaxing solutions (often lye-based), heat-styling products, alcohol based products, and even the chlorine in swimming pools. With prolonged exposures, these chemicals can really take the shine right out of your hair.

330.   Try using gel for controlling hair when you desire that "wet" effect. Apply a little gel to your hair after it's styled. When braiding, use it on all of the hair prior to braiding, or when you need your hair off your face. You may even use it on the perimeter of your hairline, where the hair is shorter.

331.   Avoid using any products on your hair that contain alcohol. Some products like mousse, hairspray and gel contain alcohol which can dry hair out. If used excessively, these products can also cause damage to your hair. Before buying or using a product, check the label to be sure it doesn't contain alcohol.

332.   Although it costs less to highlight, color or perm your hair on your own, these things are usually best handled by professionals. Home kits can damage and "fry" your hair; reversing that damage can cost a lot, and damage hair even more. A good stylist can

help you get the hair that you want without damaging it.

333.   Squeeze your hair dry with a towel after shampooing. Do not rub your towel vigorously all over your head in order to dry your hair. This ruffles the hair cuticles and causes tangling of the hair. Instead, gently squeeze separate sections of your hair to get the excess water out.

334.   Choose a hairstyle that goes well with the shape of your face. Try different styles until you find one that flatters your best features and hides the ones you do not care for. Pay attention to how people with a similar facial shape wear their hair, to get a better idea of what works and what doesn't!

335.   Clean and wash your combs and brushes weekly. Dirty tools mean dirty hair. You will undo any good you have done by washing your hair, if you use a dirty comb immediately afterwards. Many people do not pay attention to their combs. Be wary of allowing your products to fall behind the sink or toilet.

336.   If your hair is thin or overly flat, head over to your refrigerator! A mixture of egg yolk and rum can give your hair the body it needs. Simply mix the ingredients, and apply it to your hair like you would

a conditioner. Let it soak for 15 minutes, and then wash it out.

www.ingramcontent.com/pod-product-compliance
Lightning Source LLC
Chambersburg PA
CBHW060752260726
48660CB00002B/583